Emergency Evacuations:
20 Useful Lessons to Get out Fast when it Matters Most!

Table of content

Introduction

Emergency evacuation is the locomotion of the people to a safe place when they feel any threat or possibility of a threat. This emergency evacuation can be due to any natural disaster or any manmade disaster. Examples of natural disaster include earthquake, hurricane, storm etc. Manmade can be due to explosions in nuclear reactors, war, fire, collapse of the building due to structure failure, accidents etc. This emergency evacuation can be at the small level or at large level. In the case of contamination of an area where the people need to be evacuated, the people are decontaminated first. There should be a thorough planning for emergency evacuation so people and their belongings can be saved to the optimum level. This emergency evacuation has certain aspects that are needed to be understood. First of all the basics of emergency evacuation should be known, there should be adequate planning not for the only fit but also people with disability and all the family members and your friends should have complete insight how to deal with this situation and how to survive such situation. We never know when we can meet with any emergency situation but we should be prepared for such situation to prevent losses. This can be achieved with the right information from the right source. Here we are providing you with some very important information that will help you in such situations. This is not only beneficial for you but your family and all the people around you.

Chapter 01: Understand the Basics of Emergency Evacuation

Multiple reasons compel us to evacuate a building or a place. Usually, a building or place is evacuated because of danger that can be in the form of storm, earthquake, bombing, war, industrial hazards etc. a building is evacuated b following Fire Evacuation Plan. When any situation is encountered which require emergency evacuation the employees who have been made responsible for such evacuations hold the responsibility of evacuating every person in the building, ensuring shutting off every equipment that has been running and all the fire doors have been cleared.

When any emergency situation is faced it is also the duty of the Manager/ Director/ Supervisor (Alternate) or Supervisor to ensure evacuation of each and every person from the building in the appropriate timescale and at the appropriate place. It is also the duty of these authorities to notify in the case when any of the people is not evacuated or missing that was accounted to be present.

Procedure of Evacuation:

- Every alarm should be considered as emergency

- To reach the place of exit people should walk instead of running to prevent any stampede which could be disastrous later on.

- Avoid use of elevators as there is greater chance of their failure or collapse

- Any electrical equipment, water faucets, lights, heating system or gas should be off

- Shut the door when leaving a place

- Only important stuff like backpacks, purse, jackets, keys, medications etc. should be taken.

- All the instructions should be followed as directed by the emergency personnel.

- Assistance should be provided to the person in need

- Emergency instructions should listen properly without making noise

- Every door should be checked before opening so if it is hot it should not be opened and move to another exit point

- If the space between your stand point and the exit door is filled with smoke then you should travel that space while crawling

- Any missing person who should be on the list should be reported as soon as possible to the police or Emergency Coordinator.

- Inhalation of smoke can be fatal and injurious so it should be avoided.

In case of unable to evacuate:

- Search for a distant room or office that has a window

- To keep the smoke out of the room close the door as well. Any crack or gap should be filled with paper or cloth preferably wet. This will keep the smoke out of the room.

- Open the window and hang any visible piece of cloth or paper and close the window over it. If there are any drapes or shades keep them open. All these actions will alarm the rescue team that someone is inside the room.

- Wait for rescue team

- Do not go back to the building until instructed by the police /fire personnelOr Emergency Coordinator.

Evacuation of handicap or disabled people:

People who are disabled can be anyone like students, visitor or employee. This disability can be variable ranging from impairment of vision, mobility, hearing or any combination of these. The evacuation of a person with a disability with your only sole responsibility can be your very last option. For evacuation of a person with a disability, you should consider multiple options with the risk of each to yourself and to the others. Try to calm yourself and do not panic as you can create a much worse condition when there is already an emergency. You should not go for rescuing a disabled alone unless you have professional training or the person is in great need of evacuation as his life is in danger and cannot wait until the arrival of the help.

Guidelines for Emergency Classroom Evacuation

- Evacuation will be discussed by the teaching faculty at the beginning of each new class as it is their responsibility. This class should discuss the entire evacuation plan according to types of emergencies that can be encountered.

- The focus of the instructor will be towards imparting knowledge to the students about the locality of fire pulls stations, fire extinguishers and all fire exits in the very close vicinity dictated for each classroom area.

- In an attempt of evacuation, the instructor will aid all the students to safely evacuate the classroom. This task will be accomplished by guiding and commanding the students to the nearest safe location. During all this drill the instructor will also guide the students towards common assembly point. There should be proper counting of each and every student by the instructor so no student is left behind. The student will only leave the area of assembly point under command by Emergency Coordinator or Police Department unless they will not.

- It will be the responsibility of the instructor to assist students with ADA so that they can be evacuated safely from the building. If any of the students with ADA need further assistance, this must be notified to Police Department or Emergency Coordinator so that the student with ADA can be safely evacuated. No need to re-enter the building until getting any command from the rescue team.

- The students with ADA then will get aid from Police Department. All the College employees hold the responsibility of safe evacuation of all visitors and students.

- Students have to follow the evacuation process by following commands from Emergency Coordinator, Instructor, Campus Director or Program Director.

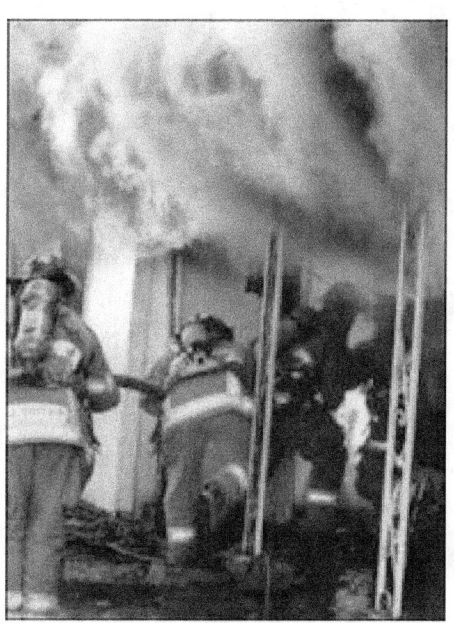

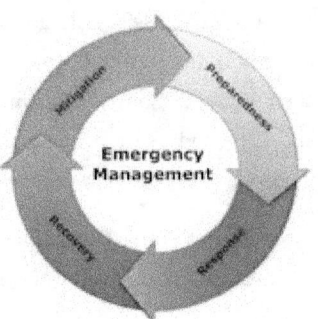

Chapter 02: Tips to Plan for Workplace Emergency and Evacuation

An emergency plan should be present as I cover all the action that needs to be followed by employers or employees for the safe evacuation of every person. Here are some tips for workplace emergency and evacuation:

- First of all, think for the worst what can happen to a building in a case of emergency then make plans according to it.

- Every action plan should be known to every person of the building.

- Involve management team and employees in your plan.

- Look at the wide varieties of emergencies that can affect a place and modify the action plan for them.

- If there is more than one work place then there should be an action plan for each work site.

- For testing of your action plan you have to implement a hazard valuation test. With this, you can see the strengths and weaknesses of your action plan.

- An action plan that is planned must include a valid system for reporting an emergency which can alarm the rescue team

- An action plan must also include a proper procedure outline covering all aspects with complete information regarding the procedure of evacuation, the route to exit and safe areas.

- There should be a proper action plan for the employees who are designated for blackout, critical plant operations, control fire extinguishers or responsible for other essential services

- Some plants that cannot be a blackout for every, emergency alarm before evacuating needed to be run.

- Name and number of people who will provide medical assistance should also be the part of an action plan with proper procedure.

- Also, there should be a site located that can give information about safe evacuation of each employee so that the authorities will have an accountable number of employees that have been evacuated.

- There should be a store on-site or off-site store that can store originals or duplicate prints of accounting annals, legal papers, your employees emergency contact registers, and other indispensable accounts

- The action plan must also have an alarming system that will be able to alarm every person of the emergency situation.

- The alarm system must be exquisite and identifiable by each employee.

- There should be a proper emergency communication system that can comprise of portable radio component

- , public speech system, or other means that can alarm the employees as well as the local rescue team.

- The alarm should be heard or seen by every employee.

- These alarms should have a backup power source so that they can even run in case of power failure.

- Tactile devices can be used for alerting employees who you know will not be able to hear an alarm.

- The action plan should be organized to prevent any confusion on the last moment.

- An action plan must also include the condition which is necessary for an evacuation.

- There should be an authorized portfolio of the plan and the designated person who will implement and command those actions. This should be known by every employee.

- All the evacuation routes and exit points should be known by every employee. Post this information on a place where every employee can see it properly.

- This plan should be in different languages o that the entire employee who does not understand English can take advantage of it.

- There should be separate action plans for people with disabilities.

- All the employees who have been designated for shutting out the system should know all the pros and cons and be able to recognize when they need to evacuate a place.

- There should be a proper system for taking into account all the employees who have been safely evacuating and who did not.

- The local rescue team can direct you the instruction for evacuation of a place.

- There are some special situations when they can direct you to stay at home and to shut electricity, gas or water. In such conditions, turn on the radio or TV and listen to the news.

- In some cases, it is the duty of the designated authority to hire people who hold the responsibility of shutting these utilities.

- In the case of fire, the best plan to evacuate is to run out of the building to the nearest safest place.

- In another case when there is an incident of toxic gas release hazard in your locality or a place farther, the best way is to keep indoor.

- The construction of the building is a very important aspect that needs to be considered during a disaster. As you may have to stay in the building with good construction in case of earth quake, storm or hurricane etc. buildings made up of steel are quite sound.

- There should be a complete list of designated people in case e of any atrocity and the entire employee should have an idea that to whom they have to listen.

- The coordinator for evacuation should know his/her duties. They should assist every individual to safety. Supervision of all areas including the emergency personnel. They should be in contact with the medical aid and local fire departments, and make sure that they are available with full equipment's in time, of need.

- There should be a proper plan for accountability of every employee that has evacuated.

- The assembly area should be properly known.

- There should be proper medical assistance aids available.

- Proper drills should be practiced for the action plan.

- Plans should be distributed among the ind

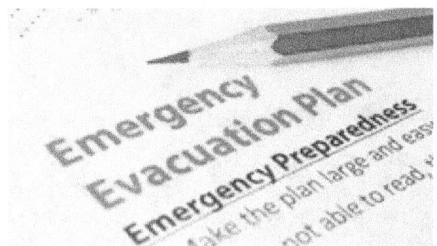

Chapter 03: Evacuation Plan for Disable Persons

The emergency action plan is devised for evacuation of every person. This plan also needs s to cover people with disability. The emergency team may not be able to count or locate the people having a disability in an emergency situation among all the other people. So, for those individuals necessary modifications are needed so that they can be assisted for their safe evacuation. This increases the chances of safe evacuation of those individuals.

Following plans should be followed for their safe evacuation:

Pre-planning (Student):

- The instructor or coordinator must have a complete insight into the capabilities and disabilities of the disabled person beforehand. So, that they can decide at what places they will need assistance.

- These people should have a complete idea about exits, halls, silos, fire alarms, fire-fighting equipment and telephones.

- These people should know any refuge place in case the will be unable to evacuate a place.

- Assistant can be designated who can assist them during an emergency.

During an emergency (Student):

- If the student is on the ground or first floor they can easily leave that place without any supervision via entitled exit route.

- Assistance can be taken from the pre-designated assistants

- People who are in wheel chairs should use elevators as their first adoption except in cases of earthquake, fire or tornado.

- If any of the people is unable to evacuate a place, they can take assistance by calling the local emergency department and can tell their location and which sort of assistance they require.

- In the case of fire or smoke which has filled a place, any local person can be alerted by waving of a light-colored cloth or a whistle.

- In the case of an earthquake, the best process is to take refuge in the nearest safest place except for the windows.

- In the case of a tornado or severe weather condition, move to the safest location as designated in the emergency plan.

- Give the advice to the person that how he/she can give you best assistance for transportation.

Pre-planning (staff members):

- It is the duty of staff member to notify them students in the beginning of each semester the plan for emergency situations and disabled students should also know their accommodations in such cases.

- Faculty will arrange volunteer students who can assist students with a disability.

- The faculty has to be familiar with exits, ramps, stairwells, emergency telephones and elevators designated for disabled people.

- They should provide proper training to the disabled student.

During an emergency (staff members):

People with wheel chairs:

- People with wheel chair and struck on the first floor can go to nearest exit route with assistance from the volunteer.

- A person with wheel chair and are struck on the second floor or higher can go to stair well with assistance from the volunteer.

- As soon as the stair well is cleared, the disabled can move to the stairs with or without assistance.

- If the disabled cannot cross the stair then the staff member must notify the emergency team outside the building to send help. There is no excuse to leave a student alone.

People with visual loss:

- They should be notified of the emergency situation by the faculty.

- The faculty have to tell them who they are and then they can assist them with the evacuation plan

- Guide them by holding their arm. Do not grasp them.

People with hearing impairments:

- Give them the notes in written so that they can know the emergency plan with clear instructions and all the exit routes.

- To alarm these individual of an emergency tap on their shoulder or turn on/ off a light.

- Indicate them the plan by gestures or in writing and then assist them.

People using crutches, canes, or walkers:

- These people need assistance for evacuation. Treat them as injured during an emergency.

- The faculty member can carry them with the help of volunteers in two-person, lock arm position or have the person sit in a chair with arms.

Non-ambulatory person:

- These people may not need assistance for walking through the ground floor.

- Approach them and ask them the best way in which they want to get carried or if the   need   any   assistance.

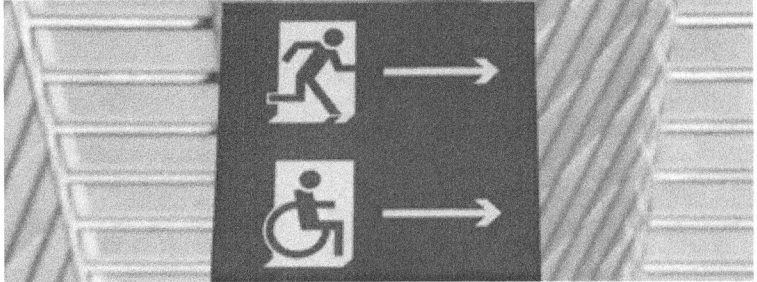

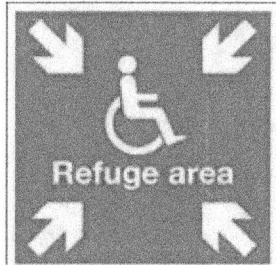

Chapter 04: Tips to Survive a Terror Attack

When any of the terror attacks is encountered, the first question that comes to mind is how to deal with it? This worry is necessary as not only the life of one but all the family members are in danger.

Many officials have implicated the act of 'run if you can' instead of to stay there and lie down or to hide at a place with mobiles on silent mode. The outline of this chapter is to define the strategies that need to be followed in such situations and to build such premises that prevent entry of terrorists.

A terrorist can implement their terror in a number of ways like intimidations of terrorism, murders, abductions, skyjackings, bombings, cyber-attacks or the usage of bio-chemical, organic, nuclear, and radiological arms which can directly or indirectly affect lives of individuals.

The people or places with high risk of terror include military and civilian government facilities, hefty cities, international airports, high-profile benchmarks, large public assemblies, water and food supply centers and their distributaries, utilities, commercial centres, mailings (different sort of chemical, biological or explosives agents can be sent through the mail). These places need pre-planned strategies to avoid nuisance.

The first point to ponder is the prevention of this attack. This can be attributed by identifying the people who can provide terror to the people. These people can be identified by keeping eye on the seven signs of terrorism which need to be identified as early as possible.

- **Surveillance**:

The very first thing to notify is to look for the people who you think monitoring a lot around a place or people. He/ she may not be taking obvious recordings with a camera or video but that can be in the form of notes, sketching diagrams, interpreting maps, or use of binoculars etc.

- **Illustration:**

Look around at the people who show much interest in army exercises, capabilities, short comings or military operations. This conversation may not be in person but can be made via text messages, phone call, Skype, emails etc.

- **Security strength evaluation:**

If you find someone having a keen interest in security strength and falls off a place or if he/ she is attempting to evaluate such strength and falls by noticing reaction time provided by a security upon breach notify it to the security services.

- **Supply chain**:

There should be accountability of the people who you think are collecting explosive materials, weapons or ammunition etc. by buying and stealing. Other necessary items to plan a terror attack may include military dresses, flight handbooks, emblems or the equipment to make them, and any other controlled items. Some terrorist manifested terror by use of fireworks and pressure cookers.

- **Suspicious person:**

Everyone has a great insight about the people living in their neighbourhood. If any of such person is identified with suspicious activity it should be notified. Such incidence can even happen at work, businesses, or anywhere. Also, there should be great awareness regarding people who cross borders out of law, board in on a ship deliberately, or hurdle ship in the harbor if you are travelling in it.

- **Trial run:**

A terrorist does plan the terror attack and to evaluate its validity they practice it. So look around the people who are moving without purposes. The terrorist also plans out escape routes, alternate exit points, the timing of arrival of security officials and time for traffic light operation. These activities needed to be evaluated and notified for safety purposes.

- **Situating assets:**

Terrorists need skilled people and ample supplies before implication of a terror attack. If any of such activity is noticed, it should be notified to the local security activists. This can be the last chance before persuasion of a terror attack.

All the officials encourage family members to take time out and practice against the act of terrors. There are three simple steps that you need to do:

- Identify your work, school, building, community emergency plan management. If you do not have any idea about theses then contact the emergency department for the plan layout.

- Keep a track record of alternative hospitals as a terror attack is manifested the nearest hospitals are busiest.

- Online resources should be sought out in such cases for managing and understanding such situations.

Terrorist activities in public places:

One of the best ways to keep your family safe is to identify these suspects. These can be prevented by correct intervention; the most impiortant6 implication is to 'look and listen'. Look for:

- Bags which are left in the public places unattended.

- People keeping surveillance of important buildings.

- People who buy force try to enter an area or premises.

- People at a place when covered with a lot of clothes.

Terrorist activities via explosive materials:

Terrorist usually implicates terrorist activities by use of explosive materials. You and your family should have a complete insight about the suspect causing such nuisance and identification of these explosives. Look for these:

- When the supplies that have been delivered are unanticipated or from someone unidentified to you

- There is no track of address and the parcel is not verified for identification

- When it has certain notifications like "Do not X-ray," "Confidential," or "Personal."

- They have wires or aluminium foils coming out of it.

- Have strange smell, look or odour.

- The address that is mention is not in relevance to the city or state

- They are of unusual size, weight for their size or are in bad condition or having odd shape

- Some form of threatening language is written over it

- If they are marked with unusual labelling

- They have been covered with extra covering or masking tapes

- There are wrong spelling of common words over the box

- It has address of someone else and is not relevant

- The tilted for the recipient is not present or is incorrect

- The specificity of the recipient is not mentioned

- The address is poorly written or typed.

Interventions during terror attack:

Some safety rules that needs to be followed by explosions include:

- Use flash light for directing the rescuers of your location.

- No unnecessary movement should be made as it can stir dust.

- Cover nose and mouth with a piece of cloth or tissue paper and breath through it.

- You can tap on wall, doors or pipes so that rescuers can hear your voice and assess your location

- Whistles can be manifested as a sign of locations.

- Shouting can be the only last asset because it can cause you to inhale a lot of dust.

- Get under study table if a lot of material is falling.

- Follow emergency plan that has been devised by the community or your family

- Do not use elevators.

- Avoid crowds, unattended vehicles.

- Do not stand in front of window, door or glass.

- Help people who need assistance.

- Keep in touch with the locals with the help of phones, radios or television.

- Keep first aid kits at home including hard caps and masks.

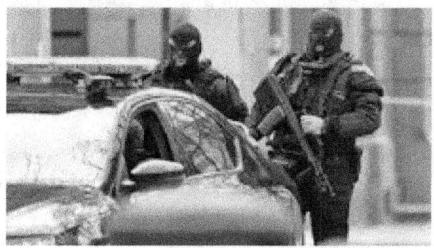

Chapter 05: Evacuation Guidelines for You and Your Family

Many emergencies compel the citizens to evacuate. When the evacuations are unavoidable the community is directed by the officials to evacuate. These can be done by media, sirens, text alerts, emails or telephone calls. Different disasters provide different time limits for evacuation like a hurricane can require one or two days but some do not give time to think so pre-planning is crucial in such cases.

This plan should include the assembly point for family union and need of supplies at the home.

Guidelines for evacuation:

- These guidelines will be necessary to follow in an attempt of evacuation.

- Make a plan for the place where the family will meet after separation. Plan more than one place in the immediate neighbourhood.

- Plan more than one route to the assembly point.

- Keep gas tank of the car full if there is need of evacuation. Also keep extra fuel as gas stations are usually shut down during emergency conditions.

- Keep a track record of an alternative route of transportation from your area to a safe one.

- Leave as early as possible to avoid trapping in worst conditions.

- Follow the routes that have been deciding before. Do not go for short cuts as they might have blocked in such situations.

- Be aware of the road conditions that you may encounter like drained roads or overpasses and broken power lines.

- Plan to take one car per family to reduce congestion and delay

- Do not go towards flooded areas.

- If there is no way for your own transportation means then plan out with family, friends and neighbours that how will you evacuate?

- Keep a radio that works with a battery and follow the instructions provided by the local emergency department. Also, listen to the local weather reports.

- Keep emergency evacuation kit with you with all necessary supplies.

- Do not leave your pets and take with you.

- Call, send a message or email any family member or friend about the location you are heading to.

- Keep all the windows, doors and chimneys closed, of your home, to secure it before leaving.

- Power off the electricity equipment. Only leave freezers and refrigerators running unless there is threat of flood.

- Turn off electricity, gas and water supply if there is a risk of damage to your home.

- Leave a letter or note adressing your location for the family and friends.

- Wear heavy shoes and full clothing for protection.

- Do ask the neighbours if they need any help.

Fire alarm evacuation tips:

Whenever you hear the sound of an n emergency alarm immediately show response according to it. These are set to prevent hazards to you and your family. This Fire Alarm System is intended to provide you with an early threatening to allow you to securely exit the constructing premises during an emergency situation.

- Don't ignore the alarm, adopting the alarm is false, or assume it is only a fire alarm test.

- Everyone must evacuate the building by way of the safest and closest exit and/ or stairway. Never use an elevator to exit during a fire alarm initiation.

- Once outside the building, move away from the building. Assemble across the street or along the sidewalk of the adjacent building.

- The anterior of the building is where the fire fighters and fire trucks will be functioning. Do not hinder their admittance to the building.

- If an event has occurred on the upper floors and glass is being gusted out of the windows, the zone below is the hazard zone where serious individual injuries will happen. Stay away from this hazard zone.

- Once outside, never re-enter the premises until you are told to do so by the fire department or Police.

Conclusion

No one expects any emergency or disaster anytime but this fact is unavoidable as they can be struck at any place at any time and to anyone. These can strike anyone. The best way to prevent these hazards is pre-planning which can be done for individuals, family members, friend or the community. These safety plans are made for the people and are therefore expected to be followed by the correct standard. These plans are different for disabled people and should be followed as such. The very crucial stand point that needs to be implicated is the correct provision of knowledge about these plans to the people so precious lives can be saved easily. All the people should have complete access to these plans and they should have command over these. Appropriate training sessions should be planned for drills so that people can easily understand these plans. One of a terrifying situation that is encountered now a days is terror attack which has created a rage all around the world. These terror attacks can be avoided by correct interventions and if struck, proper management can save lives of many people. These practices need to be launched on community levels with the involvement of every individual for optimum outcome. If all these interventions are followed, cost and lives can be saved to the optimum extent. In the end, I would like to thanks the reader for downloading this book.

FREE Bonus Reminder

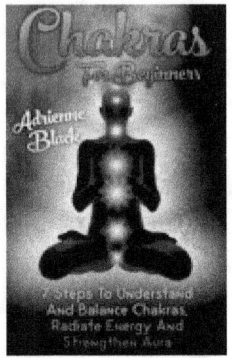

If you have not grabbed it yet, please go ahead and download your special bonus E book *"Chakras for Beginners. 7 Steps To Understand And Balance Chakras, Radiate Energy, And Strengthen Aura"*.

Simply Click the Button Below

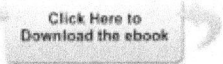

OR Go to This Page

http://lifehacksworld.com/free

BONUS #2: More Free & Discounted Books & Products

Do you want to receive more Free/Discounted Books or Products?

We have a mailing list where we send out our new Books or Products when they go free or with a discount on Amazon. Click on the link below to sign up for Free & Discount Book & Product Promotions.

=> Sign Up for Free & Discount Book & Product Promotions <=

OR Go to this URL

http://zbit.ly/1WBb1Ek